C000146182

*Lynne Robinson* is a leading Pilates specialist, whose best-selling first book with Gordon Thomson, *Body Control – The Pilates Way*, has won wide acclaim. Widely featured on TV and in magazines for her work, she is also co-author with Helge Fisher of *Mind-Body Workout*, and is presenter of Telstar's top-selling *Body Control* video, and the new *Pilates Weekly Workout*.

*Gordon Thompson*, formerly of the Ballet Rambert and London Contemporary Dance, runs the prestigious Body Control Pilates Studio in London's South Kensington. He is co-author of the original *Body Control – The Pilates Way*.

*Helge Fisher* is qualified in anatomy, physiology and holistic massage, and is an Alexander Technique teacher. The co-author with Lynne Robinson of *Mind-Body Workout*, she has been teaching Body Control Pilates for over ten years.

### Advice to the Reader

Before following any of the exercise advice contained in this book it is recommended that you consult your doctor if you suffer from any health problems or special conditions or are in any doubt as to its suitability.

# The Morning Energizer

Lynne Robinson, Gordon Thomson & Helge Fisher

PAN BOOKS

First published 1999 by Pan Books
an imprint of Macmillan Publishers Limited
25 Eccleston Place, London SW1W 9NF
Basingstoke and Oxford
Associated companies throughout the world
www.macmillan.com

ISBN 0 330 37327 7

9 8 7 6 5

A CIP catalogue record for this book is available from the British Library.

Text design by Neil Lang
Printed and bound in Belgium

# Contents

Introduction 6

The Eight Principles of the Pilates Method 7

Before You Begin 8

Checking your Alignment 9

The Position of the Pelvis and Spine 10

Breathing the Pilates Way 12

Creating a Strong Centre 14

**The Exercises**

The Morning Stretch 16

The Starfish 18

Shoulder Drops 20

Spine Curls 22

Hip Rolls 26

Early Morning Curl Ups 30

Obliques 32

The Hundred 34

The Star 38

Rest Position 42

Roll Downs 44

# Introduction

Your wake-up alarm rings, do you:

a) Think 'yippee' and leap out of bed?
b) Press the snooze button and snuggle back under the covers for that extra five minutes – which you know will make you late because you've already planned the time it takes you to get ready down to the last second?

If you answered b) then this book is for you! Initially, you might be even later for work, but it won't be long before you set that alarm for twenty minutes earlier and jump out of bed just so that you can enjoy these early morning exercises.

Designed to make you feel good and look great, there is no better way to start the day. Gentle stretches to lengthen you, deep abdominal exercises to strengthen your torso, efficient breathing to nourish and rejuvenate every cell in your body.

When every minute counts, these precise, controlled movements will ensure you make the most of your time and your body. With your mind focused, your body prepared, the day is for the taking . . .

# The Eight Principles of the Pilates Method

The exercises in this book have their origins in the work of Joseph Pilates (1880–1967). A well-proven method in existence for over seventy-five years, they also incorporate the latest techniques in both mental and physical training, offering complete body conditioning.

The programme targets the key postural muscles, building strength from within, by stabilizing the torso. The body is gently realigned and reshaped, the muscles balanced, so that the whole body moves efficiently. By bringing together body and mind and heightening body awareness, Pilates literally teaches you to be in control of your body, allowing you to handle stress more effectively and achieve relaxation more easily.

All the exercises are built around the following Eight Principles:

| | |
|---|---|
| **Relaxation** | **Co-ordination** |
| **Concentration** | **Centring** |
| **Alignment** | **Flowing movements** |
| **Breathing** | **Stamina** |

## Before You Begin

▷ The exercises should ideally be done on a padded mat.
▷ Wear something warm and comfortable, allowing free movement.
▷ Barefoot is best, socks otherwise.
▷ You may need, a firm flat pillow or folded towel, a larger pillow, a long scarf and a tennis ball.

### Please do not exercise if:

▷ You are feeling unwell
▷ You have just eaten a heavy meal
▷ You have a bad hangover or have been drinking alcohol
▷ You have taken painkillers, as it will mask any warning pains

If you are undergoing medical treatment, are pregnant or injured, please consult your medical practitioner. It is always advisable to consult your doctor before you take up a new exercise regime.

## Checking Your Alignment

Always take a moment to check that your body is correctly aligned before you start an exercise. Here is a checklist to help:

▷ Is my pelvis in neutral? See page 10.
▷ Is my spine lengthened, but still with its natural curves? Think of the top of the head lengthening away from the tailbone.
▷ Where are my shoulders? Hopefully not up around your ears! Keep the shoulder blades down into your back, a nice big gap between the ears and the shoulders.
▷ Is my neck tense? Keep the neck released and soft, the back of the neck stays long.
▷ Where are my feet? Don't forget them, for if they are misplaced it will affect your knees, hips and back. Usually, they should be hip-width apart, in parallel. Watch that they do not roll in or out!

## The Position of the Pelvis and Spine

If you exercise with the pelvis and the spine misplaced you run the risk of creating muscle imbalances and stressing the spine itself. You should aim to have your pelvis and spine in their natural, neutral positions.

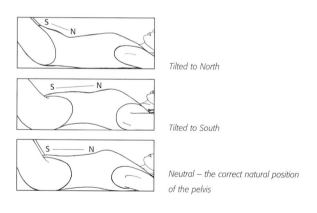

*Tilted to North*

*Tilted to South*

*Neutral – the correct natural position of the pelvis*

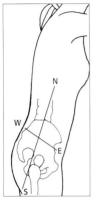 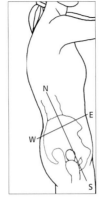 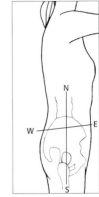

*Wrong*                    *Wrong*                    *Right*

## Breathing the Pilates Way

In Pilates we use lateral, thoracic breathing for all exercises. This entails breathing into the lower ribcage and back to make maximum use of lung capacity. The increased oxygen intake replenishes the body and the action itself creates greater flexibility in the upper body. It also works the abdominals.

To learn lateral breathing you may sit, stand or kneel, your pelvis in neutral, the spine lengthened.

Wrap a scarf around your ribcage, cross the ends over in the front and pull a little on them to feel where you are working. The idea is to breathe into the scarf, directing the breath into your sides and back, but keeping the shoulders down and relaxed, and the neck calm.

The ribs expand as you inhale, close down as you exhale.

Repeat six times but do not over-breathe or you may feel dizzy.

Breathe softly in a relaxed way.

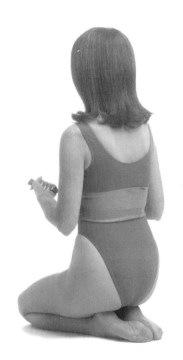

*Breathe in wide and*
*full to prepare for*
*movement*
*Breathe out as you move*
*Breathe in to recover*

## Creating a Strong Centre

Nearly all Pilates exercises involve engaging the deep postural muscles to protect the spine as you exercise. This is called 'stabilizing' or 'centring' and creates a 'girdle of strength' from which to move.

To find these deep muscles, adopt the Starting Position opposite:

▷ Breathe in to prepare and lengthen through the spine.
▷ Breathe out and engage the muscles of your pelvic floor (as if you are trying not to pass water) and hollow your lower abdominals back to your spine. Do not move the pelvis or spine.
▷ Breathe in and release.

Think of it as an internal zip which begins underneath and zips up and in to hold your lower abdominal contents in place, just like zipping up your trousers. '**Zip up and hollow**'.

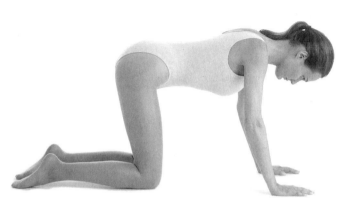

*Come onto all fours, hands beneath shoulders, knees beneath your hips. Look straight down at the floor, the back of the neck stays long, the spine maintains its natural neutral curve.*

# The Morning Stretch

### Starting Position
▷ Sit with your knees bent and the soles of your feet together.
▷ Do not bring your feet too close to you, you should be comfortable.
▷ Your pelvis should be square. You could sit with your back to a wall to check this.

### Action
▷ Breathe in to prepare and lengthen up through the spine.

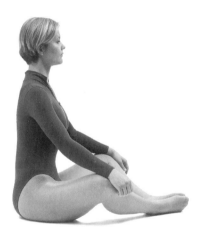

▷ Breathe out and, **zipping up the pelvic floor and hollowing navel to spine**, relax forward.

▷ Take twelve breaths, breathing into your lower ribcage and back. Relax into the stretch edging forward if you can, still hollowing. Your arms are resting in front of, your neck is long, your shoulder blades resting down into your back.

▷ After twelve breaths, slowly unfurl on the out-breath, **zipping up and hollowing**, rebuilding the spine vertebra by vertebra.

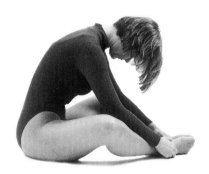

## The Starfish

**Starting Position** (this is called the **Relaxation Position**)

▷ Lie with your knees bent, feet hip-width apart and in parallel. If your chin is pointing backwards or your neck arching back use a small flat firm pillow or simply fold a towel into four, and lay it under your head to bring the face into parallel with the floor. Allow the floor to support you.

▷ Allow your body to widen and lengthen.

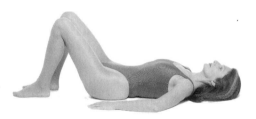

**Action**

▷ Breathe in wide and full to prepare.

▷ Breathe out, **zipping up and hollowing**, slide the right leg away from you along the floor, whilst taking the left arm above you, soft and wide, in a backstroke movement to touch the floor if you can. Do not force the arm or allow the upper back to arch. Keep the pelvis still.

▷ Breathe in, still **zipping and hollowing**, and return to the start position.

Repeat five times to each side. Take care that your pelvis stays in neutral, your shoulder blades stay down into your back and your neck stays released.

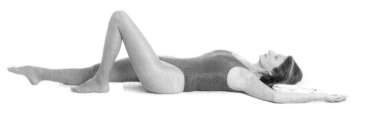

## Shoulder Drops

Lie on your back in the Relaxation Position (page 18).

▷ Raise both arms towards the ceiling directly above your
  shoulders, palms facing.
▷ Reach for the ceiling with one arm, stretch through the
  fingertips. The shoulder blade comes off the floor, then drop
  the arm back down into the floor.

Repeat ten times with each arm. Feel your upper back widening
and the tension in your shoulders releasing down into the floor.

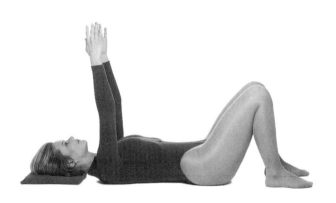

## Spine Curls

Wake up your
spine and get to
know it better –
you're going to
need it to be
both flexible
and stable
throughout
the day.

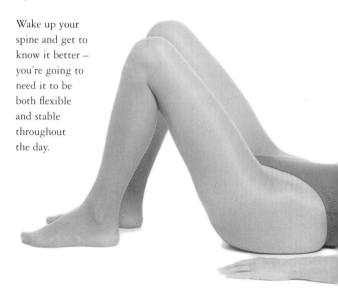

**Starting Position**

▷ Lie on your back with your knees bent, your feet about twenty centimetres from your buttocks, hip-width apart and parallel.

▷ Plant the feet firmly into the floor.

▷ If it is comfortable, take your arms above your head to rest on the floor, keeping them wider than shoulder-width, relaxed and open – your upper back must not be arched.

▷ Otherwise, leave your arms down by your sides, palms down.

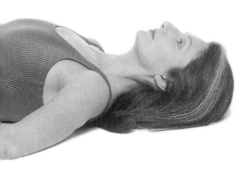

## Spine Curls (continued)

**Action**

▷ Breathe, in wide and full, to prepare.

▷ Breathe out,
   **zipping up and
   hollowing**,
   slowly and
   carefully, curl
   just the base
   of your spine
   (the coccyx, or
   tail-bone) off
   the floor. (You
   will lose the
   neutral pelvis
   position.)

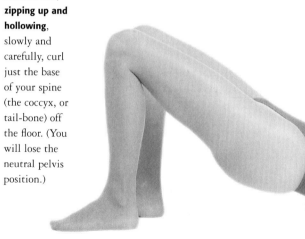

▷ Breathe in, and breathe out, still **zipping up and hollowing**, as you lower and lengthen the spine back onto the floor.

▷ Repeat, lifting a little more of the spine off the floor each time. As you lower, put down each part of the spine in sequence, bone by bone, aiming to put 'three inches' between each vertebra – the back of the ribs, the waist, the small of the back, the tailbone.

You should complete five full curls, wheeling and lengthening the spine.

▷ Take care that your back does not arch and that the tailbone stays tucked under like a whippet who has just been told off!

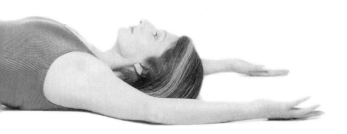

# Hip Rolls

This exercise really works the waist and the muscles along the spine.

### Please note:
Do not attempt this exercise if you have a disc-related back injury.

### Starting Position
▷ Lie on your back, arms out to the side, palms down.
▷ Your knees should be up towards your chest but in line with your hips. Your thighs will be at right angles to your body.
▷ Your feet are softly pointed.
▷ Place a tennis ball between your knees, the idea being that the ball helps to keep your knees and hips in good alignment, so it should not roll around. Gently roll your head from side to side to release the neck.

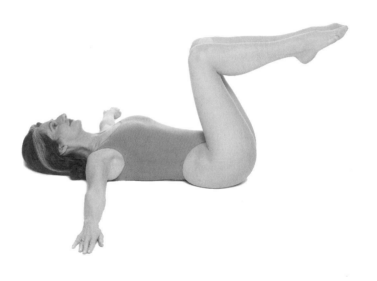

# Hip Rolls (continued)

### Action

▷ Breathe in, wide and full, to prepare.

▷ Breathe out, **zipping up and hollowing**, slowly lowering your legs toward the floor on your left side – go only a little way at first, you can go further as you become stronger. Turn your head to the right. Keep your right shoulder down on the ground, the blade down into your back. Keep the knees in-line.

▷ Breathe in, and breathe out, still **zipping and hollowing**, and use this strong centre to bring your legs back to the middle. The head returns to the middle.

Repeat ten times in each direction, moving from the strong centre.

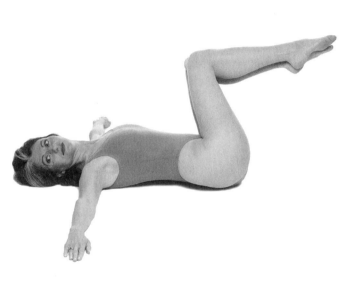

## Early Morning Curl Ups

*Lie in the Relaxation Position. Place one hand behind your head, the other hand is on your lower abdomen. This is to check that your stomach does not pop up. Your pelvis is in its neutral position.*

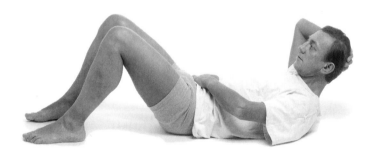

**Please note:**

Avoid this exercise if you have neck problems.

**Action**

▷ Gently release your neck by rolling the head slowly from side to side.

▷ Breathe in, wide and full, to prepare.

▷ Breathe out, **zipping up and hollowing**, soften your breastbone, tuck your chin in a little and curl up, breaking from the breastbone. Your stomach must not pop up. Keep the length and width in the front of the pelvis and the tailbone down on the floor lengthening away. Do not tuck the pelvis or pull on the neck!

▷ Breathe in and slowly curl back down.

Repeat ten times (change hands after five), being careful

▷ not to grip around the hips

▷ not to lose your neutral pelvis

▷ not to make the wrong muscles work

## Oblique Curl Ups

**Please note:**
Avoid this exercise if you have neck problems.

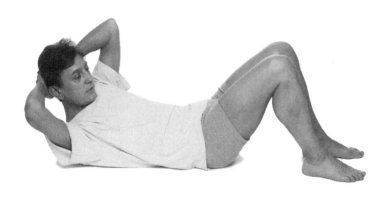

**Starting Position**

As for the previous exercise, only place both hands behind your head, the elbows staying open and placed just in front of your ears.

**Action**

▷ Breathe in wide and full to prepare.

▷ Breathe out, **zipping up and hollowing**, bring your left shoulder across towards your right knee. The elbow stays back, it is the shoulder which moves forward. Your stomach must stay hollow, the pelvis stable.

▷ Breathe in and lower.

Repeat five times to each side keeping the upper body open and the neck released.

# The Hundred

**Starting Position and Breathing Preparation.**

▷ Lie on your back in the Relaxation Position. **Zipping up and hollowing**, bring your knees onto your chest one at a time.

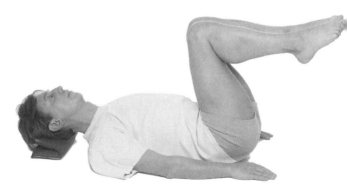

Stretch your arms down by your sides, palms down, fingers lengthening away.

▷ Breathe in wide and full into your back and sides for a count of five. Breathe out for a count of five.

▷ When you are happy with this breathing pattern, you may begin beating the arms rhythmically up and down just a few inches while breathing in for five beats, breathing out for five beats.

▷ Work up to beating one hundred times, keeping the upper body open, your shoulder blades down into your back.

## The Hundred (intermediate level)

When you have mastered the breathing, you can try the following:

**Please note:**
Please leave the head down if you have neck problems.

**Action**
▷ Breathe in wide and full to prepare.
▷ Breathe out, **zip up and hollow** and curl your head off the floor, straightening the legs into the air. Keep them in parallel.
▷ Breathe in and beat the arms for a count of five.
▷ Breathe out and beat the arms for a count of five.

Count to a hundred! Keep **zipping and hollowing**. Do not allow the legs to fall away, no daylight under your back. Keep a sense of width in the upper body, shoulder blades down into your back. Do not strain the neck.

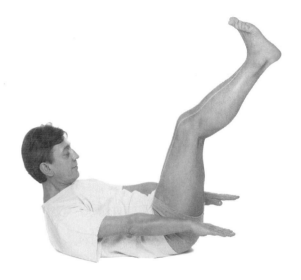

▷ When you have finished counting, lower your head, bend
  your knees, and lower them one at a time to the floor,
  **zipping and hollowing**.

## The Star

### Starting Position

▷ Lie on your front. Rest your head on your folded hands, opening the shoulders out and relaxing the upper back. If you have a back problem you may feel more comfortable with a flat pillow under your stomach.

▷ Your legs are shoulder-width apart and turned out with your feet softly pointed, unless you have suffered from sciatica, in which case leave the legs in parallel.

### Action

▷ Imagine there is a precious egg under your lower abdomen.

▷ Breathe in, wide and full, to prepare.

▷ Breathe out, **zip up and hollow** your lower abdominals as if you are trying not to crush the egg. Still breathing out, lengthen the leg before you lift it no more than ten centimetres (4 inches) off the floor, lengthening it away from the hip socket, keeping the leg straight, the foot long and the pelvis square on the ground.
▷ Breathe in and release.

Repeat three times on each side – when this is easy you may move on . . .

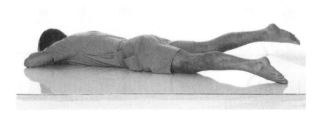

## The Star (continued)

▷ Place a small flat pillow underneath your forehead.
  Take your arms out so that you look like a star.
▷ With the next out-breath, **zip up and hollow** and
  lengthen and lift the opposite arm and leg no more than
  ten centimetres off the floor. Keep the arm soft and wide
  and the neck released, forehead down.
▷ Breathe in and release.

Repeat a further five times with each side, lengthening away from
the strong centre. Do not lift too high with the leg and keep the
head down, your neck long.

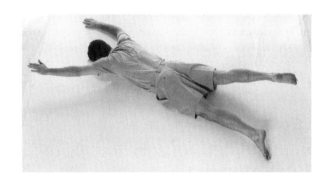

## The Rest Position

When you have finished the Star, come up onto all fours and allow the spine to lengthen out for a moment before you bring your heels together and back to sit on your heels.* Keep the knees apart and take care that you do not sit between the heels.

▷ Breathe deeply into the back of your ribcage for eight breaths. Feel the back expand and contract.

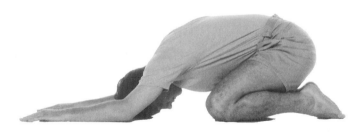

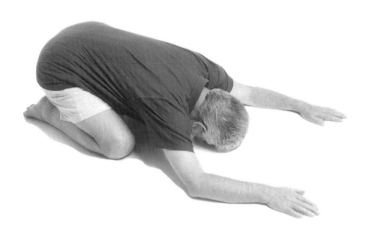

▷ After eight breaths, breathe out, **zip up and hollow**, and slowly unfurl the spine, rebuilding the column, vertebra by vertebra, until you are upright. Bring your head up last.

\* If you have a knee injury, curl up on your side in the foetal position.

# Roll Downs

### Starting Position

This position comprises excellent directions for standing well throughout the day.

▷ Stand with your feet hip-width apart and in parallel, your weight evenly balanced on both feet. Check that you are not rolling your feet in or out.
▷ Soft knees.
▷ Find your neutral pelvis position but keep the tailbone lengthening down.
▷ **Zip up and hollow.**
▷ Lengthen up through the top of your head.
▷ Shoulders widening.
▷ Arms relaxing.

### Action

▷ Breathe in, lengthen up through the spine.

- ▷ Breathe out, **zip up and hollow**, bend your knees slightly.
- ▷ Drop your chin onto your chest and allow the weight of your head to make you slowly roll forward, head released, arms hanging, centre strong, knees soft.

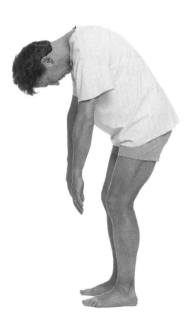

## Roll Downs (continued)

▷ Breathe in as you hang, really letting your head and arms hang.

▷ Breathe out, **zipping and hollowing**, as you drop your tailbone down, directing your pubic bone forward. Rotate your pelvis as you slowly come up to standing tall, rolling through the spine bone by bone.

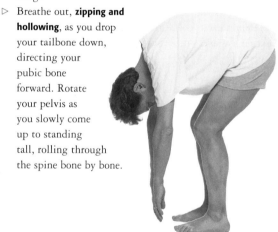

Repeat six times, wheeling the spine and making sure that you keep central.

**Please note:**
If you have a back problem, you may wish to do this exercise against a wall – stand about forty-five centimetres (eighteen inches) from the wall and lean back into it, the knees are bent so that you look like you are sitting on a bar stool.

**These fantastic Pilates books are all available from your local bookshop, or by sending a cheque or postal order as detailed below.**

**Body Control – The Pilates Way**  0 330 36945 8  £7.99  pb
The original best-selling manual taking Pilates out of the studio and into the home
**Mind–Body Workout**  0 330 36946 6  £12.99  pb
A fresh approach to exercise combining Pilates and the Alexander Technique

*Pilates Through the Day*
A series of mini-books to help your body make the most of every day
**The Morning Energizer**  0 330 37327 7  £2.99  pb
**The Desk Reviver**  0 330 37328 5  £2.99  pb
**The Evening Relaxer**  0 330 37329 3  £2.99  pb
**Off to Sleep**  0 330 37330 7  £2.99  pb

**Pilates – The Way Forward**  0 330 37081 2  £12.99  pb
Coming in April 1999, a whole new range of exercises to get you fit, keep you supple and safely work to remedy your body's problems

Book Services By Post, PO Box 29, Douglas, Isle of Man IM99 1BQ.
Credit card hotline 01624 675137. Postage and packing free.

For further information on books, videos, workshops, equipment and clothing, send an SAE to Body Control Pilates Ltd, PO Box 238, Tonbridge, Kent TN11 8ZL.
For a list of Pilates teachers and teacher training programmes, send an SAE to The Body Control Pilates Association, 17 Queensbury Mews West, South Kensington, London SW7 2DY.

Regular information updates appear on the Body Control Pilates website at www.bodycontrol.co.uk